Autism

Teach Your Autistic Children Hygiene Skills To Help Them Live A Clean, Healthy And Happy Life

Nancy Perez

Table of Contents

Introduction

Thank you for purchasing the book, "Autism: Teach Your Autistic Children Hygiene Skills To Help Them Live A Clean, Healthy And Happy Life".

As a parent of an autistic child, it can be quite daunting to teach your child hygiene skills. We know that an autistic child's idea of hygiene can be very different than the world's idea of the same. It is unconventional and in many cases makes them feel anxious.

This book will show you the most common hygiene problems that autistic children face. And provide practical solutions that you as a parent can implement to teach personal hygiene to your autistic child in a simple and effective way.

The key is to take matters slowly. Introduce personal hygiene lessons to your children in steps that they can manage. Describe each step to them. Help them remember by providing visual aids.

I hope this book helps you teach your children the hygiene skills that will help them live a clean, healthy and happy life.

Happy reading!

Hygiene Problems Your Autistic Child May Face

Helping Your Autistic Child Understand Hygiene Problems

Proper personal hygiene starts at home. Parents play an important role in making sure their autistic child knows basic, important personal hygiene. They can be the perfect role models for their child by doing and showing their child how they do good personal hygiene habits. Autistic children mimic what they see. If they see their parents regularly showering, brushing teeth, and washing hands, they'll learn these habits fast and easy. Most importantly, they'll learn that hygiene is important.

Start teaching personal hygiene at an early age. Frequent reinforcements about personal hygiene will help autistic children learn more. Giving lots of encouragement and praise for accomplishing hygiene tasks will also help.

Parents can explain to their autistic child that keeping a clean body is healthy. As an example, they can remind their child what bacteria and germs can do if someone does not wash hands before eating or after going to the toilet.

Basic, daily personal hygiene is about washing hands, keeping the body neat and clean, and covering the mouth when sneezing or coughing. There is a social element to dealing with personal things though. Here are the most common hygiene problems that autistic children may face. Parents can cite these problems when helping their autistic child understand the importance of personal hygiene habits.

Oral Hygiene

Practicing good oral hygiene is important at any age. Brushing teeth twice a day and regular flossing are important if parents want their autistic child to avoid tooth decay, bad breath, and gum problems. Parents also need to maintain regular dental appointments for their autistic child.

Body Hygiene

Good body hygiene is also important at any age. Washing and bathing regularly keep off dirt and bacteria which feed on human sweat, dead skin cells, and other bodily fluids causing bad body odor. Changing clothes and underwear regularly is part of good body hygiene too. Bad odor-causing bacteria live in soiled and smelly clothes.

When autistic children reach puberty, parents should teach them to use antiperspirant deodorant. Sweat glands in their armpit and genital area develop, increasing their chances of getting bad body odor. Allowing them to choose their own brand and scent can encourage them to use deodorants.

Toilet Hygiene and Habit

Teaching autistic children to use the toilet and helping them establish toilet hygiene are challenging tasks to go through. It takes longer for them to learn how to use a toilet than with normal children resulting in many autistic children using a toilet at a late age.

Personal Grooming

Personal grooming is more of a social reason rather than a physical one as to why autistic children should learn how to practice them. The thought of teaching them however, is daunting. Nonetheless, it is still proper to let them understand the importance of being and smelling clean, having a neat appearance, and looking nice. Enabling them to look their best can increase their confidence and may provide them with a healthy social life.

If these good personal hygiene habits are dealt with and established at an early age, they become the best foundation for good personal hygiene during teenage years. Parents with honest, open communication with their child will find it easier to discuss personal hygiene problems that occur in teenagers.

Helping Your Teenage Autistic Child Understand Hygiene Problems

Autistic children need extra care and help with personal hygiene when they reach adolescence. It is a time when the body changes, which means hygiene habits need to change and adapt, too. Parents need to help their teenage autistic son to learn how to properly shave. Parents also need to help their teenage autistic daughter to learn how to manage monthly periods, use a tampon or pad, and hygienically dispose it. It's also important to explain to autistic teenagers why certain personal hygiene should be done because they will not be able to fully understand social rules, or the reasons behind them.

The Importance of Good Personal Hygiene

Staying healthy physically involves being clean all the time. For example, washing hands, although simple as it is, is an effective and proven way of avoiding sickness and fighting off germs.

Staying healthy socially, also involves being clean all the time. Autistic children can gain confidence if they look and smell presentably well, enabling them to fit in with the crowd.

Teaching Your Autistic Child Proper Personal Hygiene

Teenagers need extra time in the bathroom. They take a bit longer (than normal kids) to accomplish hygiene tasks such as shaving or changing a tampon. Parents can help by giving them more privacy and being patient.

Autistic children need extra support with their personal hygiene, but discussing the subject with them is challenging. Learning style and ability are factors that need to be considered when thinking of teaching them good personal hygiene habits. It is vital to know how they learn important things in life.

In order for autistic children to easily learn personal hygiene, consider breaking them into small step-by-step tasks. If they are already in the habit of keeping a daily routine, that's a good thing because it'll be easier to introduce hygiene. Writing tasks in a scheduled format can also help autistic children to remember when to do their personal hygiene tasks.

Teaching Your Autistic Child to Use the Toilet

Learning and establishing good toilet habits and hygiene is not easy for autistic children. As mentioned in the previous chapter, it takes longer for them to learn how to use a toilet than normal children. For parents, it can help simplify the task by breaking it down into small parts and teach them to children one step at a time.

Steps for Teaching Your Autistic Child to Use the Toilet

The same steps in teaching children how to use a toilet are applied to autistic children as well. Aside from more time and patience, teaching them requires extra strategies and teachings that are suited to their needs.

In addition, it is important for parents, before teaching an autistic child to use a toilet, to realize first that cooperation and communication with their child is the key. It is also helpful to view toilet training as a chain of small links. Parents can start by familiarizing an autistic child with a toilet, its purpose, and how it is used.

Dealing With Challenges about Teaching Toilet Training

Changes

Autistic children are often attached, at a high level, to their activities, hobbies, tasks, and routines. They are not welcoming of any changes in their daily lives, which makes toilet training more challenging. Here are some tips to make it more bearable for both children and parents:

- Stay positive and calm. Autistic children are not fully aware of emotional responses and facial expressions. Changes in them can stress children out because they will have difficulty understanding the situation. If there is no progress after five minutes of sitting on a toilet, stop immediately and resume the next day.

  Never force autistic children to go to the toilet. Let them learn at their own pace. When they're ready, parents will surely know. In the meantime, provide encouragement and gentle reminders.

- Use a toilet training seat instead of a potty trainer. This lessens the number of changes autistic children have to go through in the process of toilet training.

- Teach children to use picture cards, nonverbal signs, or single words to indicate their need to go to the toilet. Whatever they choose, use it as the only reference to toilet. Changes in image or word association can confuse them and disrupt their toilet training tasks.

Sensory Processing Disorder (SPD)

Sensory Processing Disorder (SPD) is a disorder that often accompanies autism. In short, there is an overload of senses in an autistic child's brain, making it hard for them to focus on a task. It also makes them feel many sensations all at once, affecting the simplest activities that need to be accomplished. Here are some tips to avoid sensory overload during toilet training:

- Use a foot stool or get a child to wear socks in the bathroom to avoid the cold floor.

- Explain the noisy flushing sound of the toilet to a child, how and why it happens.

- Use a wooden training seat to avoid the cold ceramic toilet seat.

Behavior and Health Problems

Toilet habits of autistic children are sometimes associated with health and behavior problems. They may express fear of going to and using the toilet, continually flushing it, stuffing it with various materials, or smearing feces on walls. Here are some things to consider why any of these are happening:

- In a week, monitor the number of times an autistic child soils or wets the bed. Look for patterns. The next time this is about to happen again, bring the child to the toilet.

- Seek the help of doctors who work with autistic children. There could be a health or psychological reason why autistic children are acting the way they do about toilet training and hygiene. A child's lack of response to it could mean constipation, urinary tract infection, or other health and psychological problems.

- If no progress is visible, take a break from toilet training. Resume again after at least three months. This is not failure. It simply means a child is not ready yet.

Strategies for Teaching Toilet Hygiene and Habits

Visual aids, rewards, and encouragements can help autistic children learn toilet hygiene and habits.

Visual Aids and Schedules

Most autistic children are visual learners. They learn things based on what they can read or see. Picture or word cards are helpful in this strategy. Visual schedules, a list of tasks with accompanying pictures, are also helpful in telling children when to do their tasks.

Rewards and Encouragements

Use positive reinforcements and rewards whenever a child accomplishes part of a task. Use descriptive praises, nonverbal praises, favorite activities, favorite foods, or star stamps or stickers for every accomplishment or challenge. Once progress is made, stick to descriptive and nonverbal praises only.

Teaching Your Autistic Child Oral Hygiene

Oral Health Problems in Autistic Children

Autistic children experience oral health issues at a rate almost similar to normal children. It's because giving them proper oral care is difficult due to behavioral and communication problems. Here are the most common oral health problems in autistic children:

Tooth Decay

Tooth decay, or dental caries, is caused by sugar-feeding bacteria. In autistic children, a major risk of getting tooth decay is through prolonged bottle-feeding. Many of them continue to bottle-feed until the age of 4 or 5. Delays in oral-motor skills are seen to be the contributing factor.

Gum Disease

Gum disease is attributed to sensory overload in autistic children. Many do not want to brush their teeth because they do not like the sensation of bristles brushing on their gums.

Delays in Tooth Eruption

Autistic children experience delays in growth and eruption of newly developed teeth due to gingival

16

enlargement, or an increase in the size of gums. Gingival enlargement is caused by prolonged intake of Phenytoin, an anti-seizure drug often prescribed to children with Autism.

Injury and Trauma to the Mouth

Speaking of seizures, autistic children are prone to them. As a result, autistic children are at high risk of getting injuries or trauma to the mouth while experiencing seizures.

Oral health is important for autistic children, too. It is part of their general well-being. In fact, in recent years, a clear connection between overall physical health and oral health has been proven by medical research and studies.

Damaging Oral Habits

Damaging oral habits in autistic children include tongue thrusting, teeth-grinding, pica, and injury-causing behaviors such as lip-biting. Pica on the other hand, involves eating nonfood items.

Strategies for Teaching Oral Hygiene to Your Autistic Child

Making a difference in an autistic child's oral health is slow and difficult in the beginning. However, with the right determination, invaluable rewards and positive results are sure to be achieved. Here are some helpful strategies on how to teach oral hygiene to an autistic child.

Be a Good Role Model

Parents should show autistic children that they brush their teeth, too. This can build curiosity in a child until they show interest and act on their own. Once they show interest, brush teeth together. It is also important to explain to them why oral hygiene is necessary.

Use Other Options

Autistic children might not like the sensation of brushing at first, so be creative. Parents can use a clean wash cloth at first until children are accustomed to the sensation of something touching their gums and teeth. After that, they can transition to child-size toothbrush with soft bristles. Do not add in toothpaste yet. Again, allow children to get accustomed to the new sensation of a toothbrush and only after that, can toothpaste be added. Allow children to pick their toothpaste as well, preferably a mild-flavored one.

Establish a Daily Routine

It is important for autistic children to continue brushing every day. If they miss out even just for one day, they might become uncooperative the next time they are told to brush their teeth again.

Introduce Each Step One at a Time

Transitions are better when they are slower for autistic children. Take for example the introduction of a new toothbrush and toothpaste to them, as mentioned above. Do not force one step in the process. Allow children to get accustomed to each one until they are ready for the next.

Make the Process Friendlier

For autistic children with favorite objects, a book or toy for example, bringing them along while learning how to brush their teeth can be helpful. It can create a friendly environment as they learn how to brush their teeth. A friendly environment can reduce anxiety and increase compliance during the learning process.

Use Visual Aids

Because many autistic children are visual learners, using visual aids can help them understand the importance of oral hygiene and the steps involved in it. Include pictures of dentist's offices or clinics to build familiarity.

Visit a Dentist's Office, but Not to Set an Appointment

In relation to familiarity, take practice visits to the dental clinic before actually setting up an appointment. It is important for autistic children to get used to their environment before they become comfortable in them. This lessens tantrums and anxiety attacks. Again, slow transition is the best.

Remember, autistic children can only learn proper oral hygiene with gentle repetition, persistence, familiarity, and reduction in potential sensory overload that they might experience while brushing their teeth or having a visit to a dentist's clinic.

Teaching Your Autistic Child to Take a Shower

Helping Your Autistic Child Establish a Bathing Routine

Taking a shower is mostly a problem area with autistic teenagers than it is with younger children. As with any hygiene habit, it is important to start early in order to establish them onto a child. Here are tips on how to teach your autistic child to take a shower.

- Parents should organize and introduce a schedule. Write it on a sheet of paper and post it on the bathroom door or a child's room in order for it to serve as a constant reminder.

- Parents should use bath toys or other items that can help autistic children take a shower or go to the bathroom. Even older kids who bring their much-loved items in the bath are enjoying showers more. Aside from bath toys, parents can allow bubble baths and soap "paints".

- Parents should never force autistic children to take a shower every day. In fact, it is not necessary for children to bathe daily. However, if there are sanitary reasons, or special medical requirements, daily bathing is allowable. In such a case, parents should reduce anxiety levels and make bath time

21

comfortable. Use positive reinforcements or nonverbal rewards.

- Otherwise, parents can use a clean washcloth to clean autistic children on a daily basis. Make sure a child is already accustomed to using a washcloth. A sponge can also be used. Slowly introduce different kinds of washing materials to children before making them use such.

- Autistic children are often scared of big shower heads. Parents can use a flexible shower hose instead. One of the biggest obstacles in bathing for autistic children is their fear of hair washing. A flexible shower hose can help them get over their fear by giving them control of the situation. Allow them to handle the flexible shower hose on their own, but guide them gently.

- Some children are altogether afraid of taking a shower, but would love to swim. Parents can take advantage of this opportunity to bathe their children. Other times, children don't want to get wet, but love to play with sprinklers. Parents can also take advantage when this happens.

By the time autistic children have already established a routine for taking baths, parents expect them to be more responsible for keeping themselves clean. However, given their situation, parents can't help but worry. Added to the worry, children oftentimes, insist on doing it on their own. What should a parent do?

Typically, autistic children want to bathe on their own at school age. Here, they start to show personal hygiene independence. However, parents should be around to supervise the shampoo and conditioner parts of the shower. In other words, guide children through the hair washing parts, which call for patience, lots of it. At the same time, continue helping children in ways that are almost unnoticeable to them like starting the water, or passing the shampoo. This way, they still feel in control, lessening anxiety. If they want to have privacy, check on them from time to time to make sure they are cleaning themselves properly.

There's no absolute limit to when parents should allow their autistic children to bathe on their own. However, when it happens, teach children important shower and bath safety issues. This includes reminders about slippery floor, or instructions on how to regulate water temperature.

Other Hygiene Tips For Your Autistic Child

Aside from the previous personal hygiene habits, here are other hygiene tips for your autistic child. It is important mainly because it's a way to protect children from illness.

The Basics

The most basic form of personal hygiene is washing hands. Teach children to wash their hands

- before preparing, handling, and eating food

- after using the toilet

- after gardening

- after handling animals

- and after touching objects with blood or dirt.

Infectious illnesses such as gastroenteritis and colds, are mostly caught when children get germs on their hands and then they put it in their mouths. Illnesses can also be caught when other people with dirty hands touch the food that children eat. It's always important to keep clean hands, especially if children handle food all the time. Here are some tips to teach autistic children when washing their hands:

- If a child is not used to using soap, use a natural alternative. Choose a mild-scented one.

- Use soft-bristled brush to clean under nails.

- For children with fear of getting wet, use alcohol-based hand sanitizers.

- Create a fun hand washing environment by teaching them to sing while washing their hands.

Aside from these, teach children to

- be careful not to sneeze or cough on other people

- throw used tissues or anything that might have germs on them

- clean or wipe things that have been touched immediately after coughing or sneezing

- use protection when there is a risk of contagious infection

Food Handling

Children are at risk of food poisoning if they accidentally eat contaminated food, which is food with harmful germs in it. Vomiting, abdominal cramps, stomach pain, and diarrhea are tell-tale signs that a child has ingested contaminated food.

To avoid food poisoning in autistic children,

- Teach them to always clean their hands before they eat or prepare food. If there are open wounds or cuts on hands, cover it with waterproof bandage. Use colored or printed ones, so children will not worry or fear possible wounds in the future.

- Teach them to maintain a clean work area when preparing food. Teach them to wear protective clothing as well.

- Teach children to prepare raw and cooked foods separately. It is also important to teach them to use separate utensils, knives, and other food preparation utensils for different kinds of food. Raw foods are often carriers of harmful germs and bacteria.

- Teach children to wash raw foods such as fruits and vegetables, with clean water before eating them.

Blood Safety

Aside from infections caused by dirty hands and contaminated food, there are also infections that can be passed through blood contact from one person to another. And although parents will do their best to avoid their child ever seeing any blood, it is wise to teach them how to keep themselves safe. At the same time, it is also good to teach children how to handle situations when there is sight of blood. This prevents escalating anxiety levels if they accidentally cut or hurt themselves.

Here are some tips to teach children how to handle blood:

- Teach them how to seek immediate help when they injure themselves.

- Teach them not to panic at the sight of blood.

- Teach them not to touch other people's blood. If this is unavoidable, teach your child how to wear protective gloves when handling other people's wounds or injuries.

Hygiene during Travel

Traveling can disrupt children's personal hygiene routines. To make sure that they keep up with their routines, parents can:

- Bring their favorite items that they use for brushing, bathing, and all their other hygiene essentials.

- Bring their hygiene schedules and visual aids, so they still have all the references they need.

Hygiene for Girls

Here are some hygiene tips for your teenage autistic daughter:

- Teach girls not to put anything inside their genital area. Its delicate skin inside is highly sensitive and any object inserted in it can provide easy access to infection-causing germs.

- Teach girls to wash their genital area on the outside only. It can naturally clean itself on the inside.

Hygiene for Boys

Here are some hygiene tips for your teenage autistic son:

- Teach boys to wash their genital area gently

- Teach boys never to force the foreskin of their genital area away from the tip or glans. It can damage both the foreskin and the glans.

Getting Your Autistic Child to Change Clothes

Getting dressed and changing clothes can be difficult for autistic children. However, it's an important skill, so it is crucial to teach them how to do it on their own and why they have to do it. Practice, persistence, and patience are the keys in getting autistic children to do this skill.

Where to Start

Oftentimes, autistic children do not want to change clothes simply because they like what they're wearing or they do not like the other options that they see in their closets. Other times, the difficulty of removing clothes and putting them on makes children avoid the task. Parents can start by building awareness in their children that clothes have to be changed in order for the body to be clean. Make them realize that it's easy if it is done properly and in a calm manner. To make the habit fun and easy, give names to clothing, especially the favorite ones. It can also help if there is a limited choice of clothes that are easy to change into such as:

- Soft, comfortable clothes that are easy to wear and move in

- Clothes with pictures on the front to help children distinguish between front and back

- Clothes with Velcro or other fasteners that can be easily removed and attached back on

- Elastic-waisted or stretchable pants

It can be tempting to help children change clothes whenever they find it difficult. However, it is important to let them work it out for themselves in order for them to gain independence in their hygiene. The best help parents can give is to cheer them on as they try their best. Parents should only step in to help when children really need it.

Tips for Getting Your Child to Change Clothes

Children are most likely to cooperate if parents are supportive and positive. Giving a lot of praise will be helpful, even when children mistakenly wear their clothes backwards. Here are some practical tips to help parents to get their children to change clothes:

Choose Appropriate Clothes

- Foremost, teach children the difference between clean and dirty clothes. Teach them to put dirty clothes in the hamper and get clean clothes from the closet or drawers. Teach them not to wear clothes from the laundry hamper.

- Teach children to wear weather-appropriate clothes by asking them how they feel. For example, they might be cold or hot. Asking them about whether it's sunny or raining outside is also a good way to help them choose clothes.

- Allow children to choose their own clothes by guiding them to consider factors such as activities and weather. For example, if children are going to the beach, don't make them wear jackets.

Make Changing Clothes Easier

Foremost, teach children how to undress properly. It's actually easier than getting dressed and if children think that it's easy, they'll look forward to changing clothes more often.

- As mentioned earlier, provide children with clothes that have pictures on the front. This way, they'll know how to get into their clothes.

Give Them Some More Time

- Time is always an issue with autistic children. Considering they do things differently, and it takes them longer, give them more time when they change clothes. Never set a time limit.

- Practicing can always help shorten dressing time because children get accustomed to the task.

Why Autistic Children Need to Change Clothes

For autistic children, there is more to changing clothes

than just getting dressed. It builds a sense of achievement, independence, confidence, and an established personal hygiene routine. Teaching children to master this skill offers them more than just clean clothes. It also:

- Helps children raise their awareness in the environment as they dress depending on weather conditions, occasions, and activities

- Helps children widen their vocabulary as they learn to name clothes, their types, sizes, and colors

- Helps children build their cognitive, gross motor, and fine motor skills

- Helps children have more patience and focus as they concentrate on accomplishing the task

Getting Your Autistic Child a Haircut

Getting autistic children to have their haircut is probably the most difficult task yet. Considering autistic children are highly sensitive, they find haircuts scary and stressful. They might not like the feel of the cold scissors on their ears, or the sound of it. They might not like to see their hair fall on the floor or on their clothes. There are just too many reasons. Here are some tips to make haircuts less stressful for both parent and child:

- Use towels, hair cutting sheet or cape to cover a child during a haircut. Some children might find it difficult or annoying when hair falls down on their arms, shoulders, face or clothing.

- Do not force children to sit still, but teach them the benefits of getting haircuts. This way, they can behave long enough, usually in just a few minutes only, to get the job done.

- Avoid after school haircuts or when a child is sick or tired. Cut hair when a child is feeling calmer and less overwhelmed. However, it is important to set a regular schedule for haircuts and to be consistent with it.

- Autistic children might get scared with the sound of snapping scissors or buzzing hair clippers. If a child has a favorite song, try to sing together while the haircut process is ongoing. It can drown the buzzing or snapping sounds. If a child is comfortable using ear plugs, use them instead.

- Many autistic children also do not like the scent of shampoos and conditioners. Use unscented ones if planning to wash a child's hair before cutting. However, since many autistic children do not like washing their hair, dry cutting is recommended. It's also easier.

- Allow children to hold their favorite objects while their hair is cut. It can make them happy, which creates a fun environment for hair cutting.

- Use short sentences or visual aids to explain to a child the process of hair cutting. Parents can also take pictures while the process in on-going. Children meanwhile, can be allowed to take pictures of the items that will be used to cut their hair. This way, it preoccupies their mind and takes off any fear they feel.

- Focus on cutting a child's hair, but do not rush. Children might become overwhelmed with too many movements around them. Take it slowly, at the child's pace, while praising him through the process. It might be helpful to offer verbal rewards whenever a portion of hair is cut.

- Purchase a good-quality haircutting kit. Look for a

kit with scissors that have blade guards. Good quality kits make the job easier and quicker to finish.

After the haircut is done, parents should show their admiration for their child's new appearance. They should also be vocal about the new look they see. For example, tell their child how beautiful or handsome they look because of the new hairstyle. At the same time, this opportunity can be used to teach children how to comb their hair while they look in the mirror to check out their new do.

Conclusion

Thank you again for purchasing this book!

I hope this book was able to help you learn the techniques on how to teach your autistic children hygiene skills.

The next step is to use the solutions that you have read in this book and start teaching your children the basic hygiene skills that will help them live a clean, healthy and happy life.

Finally, if you found value in this book, then I'd like to ask you for a favor. Would you be kind enough to leave a review for this book on Amazon? It would be greatly appreciated!

Thank you and good luck!

Preview of "Autism: Simple And Inexpensive Natural Autism Therapies"

It can be quite a challenge to take care of a child with special needs. This challenge is compounded with the medication that your child may require to take as part of their treatment. In addition to burning a hole in your pocket, artificial medicines come with their own set of potential side-effects that can harm your child.

This book contains information about the natural therapies that can be used by parents to manage the symptoms of autism in their child. These natural therapies are relatively inexpensive compared to the prescribed medication. Some of these therapies might require professional therapists but they will be relatively cheaper compared to the traditional way of treating autism.

And since these therapies are natural they are completely safe and pose no harm to your child. Using a therapy such as Nutritional Therapy that focuses on a good diet will actually improve the health of your child. And these therapies can even be used together with the existing medications if any without having side-effects.

Nutritional Therapy

An autistic child may feel hungry but not be able to

communicate their needs. So it's important that as a parent you can understand the nutritional needs of your child.

It has been found that almost all autistic children have some form of nutritional deficiency and intolerance to certain foods. This can cause some gastric discomfort to the child as well if not taken care of.

Nutritional therapy is supposed to help improve the functioning of your child's mind and body to the best levels possible. The benefit of having this therapy in addition to the medications and other therapies is that it enhances the response of the child to such treatments.

To proceed with nutritional therapy requires a collaboration with a good dietitian to bring out a good diet plan that can take care of any nutritional deficiencies including the lack of vitamins and minerals, food intolerances and potential gastrointestinal issues.

Many autistic children can have a lack of essential vitamins, minerals and fatty acids that can reduce the efficient working of the body and mind. This can make the child irritable, have no concentration, feel depressed or anxious, lose sleep or appetite. One of the easiest ways to improve upon this is to add a good multi-vitamin and omega-3 fatty acid supplement to the diet of the child. Please make sure that these supplements are free from any artificial coloring or additives. If the child has trouble having the supplements in pill form they are also usually available as liquids that can be mixed in the food.

There are many types of diets that you can research about in details such as:

- GFCF Diet – Gluten Free Casein Free Diet

This diet involves avoiding foods that contain gluten such as bread and bakery products as well as those that contain casein such as dairy products.

- SCD Diet – Specific Carbohydrate Diet

This diet only allows consumption of carbohydrates that are easy to digest such as nuts, vegetables and fruits. All complex forms of carbohydrates such as bakery products, pasta, grains and processed foods are avoided.

- GAPS Diet – Gut and Psychology Syndrome Diet

The GAPS diet is derived from the SCD diet and involves replacing foods that are difficult to digest with foods that are simple to digest and contain a lot of nutrients.

- LO Diet – Low Oxalate Diet

This diet aims to avoid foods that can produce oxalate that can crystallize under situations and cause damage to the tissue.

- BE Diet – Body Ecology Diet

This diet attempts to maintain the ecology of the body in

balance. This involves using cultured foods, improving the quality of foods that one consumes especially fats and oils and significantly decreasing carbohydrates and sugars in the diet.

A well prepared diet for an autistic child can help reduce a lot of symptoms such as problems in speech, attention and focus, language, hyperactivity, rashes, digestion, diarrhea, constipation, fatigue, aggression, etc.

So every parent with an autistic child should learn more about the diet and nutrition that they feed their child every day. This will help you make the correct decisions when it comes to feeding your child.

Generally try to consume organic fruits, vegetables and meat. Also avoid processed foods, sugary and salty foods and foods that contain artificial colors and flavors.

Music Therapy

Music therapy is the usage of music to bring about a change in the behavior of people especially children being treated for autism.

Music therapy is carried out in sessions by a music therapist. These sessions are planned and executed based on the individual needs of each child.

Music therapy can involve playing musical instruments, listening to music, singing and being involved in action songs.

The therapy sessions are tailored specific to each autistic child because what may be good and positive for one child may be perceived as negative by another child.

There are several benefits to using music therapy with your autistic child.

There will be a significant improvement in the social development of your child once he starts learning a musical instrument. This is because he can interact with the therapist using the instrument as a means of communication. Since the music sessions are filled with fun and motivation they can help the child become more socially active and learn to interact with other people.

Music therapy can improve the speech of your child as well as comprehension skills. This is because an autistic child will be more open to sounds than speech and the use of sounds will help improve both verbal and non-verbal communication.

Autistic children who attend music therapy sessions have good improvements in their behavior. They are seen to focus better in activities and also show reduction in symptoms like aggression and anxiety.

Since music sessions are a fun activity, it is easy for the child to continue with the therapy sessions without it feeling like work. And the more sessions the child participates in, the better is the effect of the therapy.

Calm music such as those used for meditation can help reduce anxiety and panic attacks among autistic children.

Check out the rest of **Autism: Simple And Inexpensive Natural Autism Therapies** on Amazon.

Check Out My Other Books

Below are some of my other books that are popular on Amazon. Alternatively, you can visit my author page on Amazon to see other books written by me.

Autism: Simple And Inexpensive Natural Autism Therapies To Help Your Autistic Child Live A Calm And Healthy Life

Reverse Diabetes: A Step by Step Guide to Reverse Diabetes and Free Yourself from Stress, Anxiety, and Pain

www.ingramcontent.com/pod-product-compliance
Lightning Source LLC
Chambersburg PA
CBHW061801280526
45787CB00003BA/1443